Introduction

Type 2 diabetes is a cardiovascular disease and around 80% of those affected will die of coronary heart disease, stroke or peripheral vascular disease, many prematurely. The risks are magnified in individuals who have developed diabetic renal disease (nephropathy), which is also the single most common cause of chronic renal failure and need for dialysis in many countries in western Europe and the US. Records kept in Europe since 1970 show that the numbers of new patients developing end-stage renal disease are increasing exponentially. The situation is even more alarming in the US, where 40–50% of new dialysis cases are patients with diabetes. The large increase in prevalence of type 2 diabetes in recent decades, coupled with improvements in cardiovascular protection, will result in cases of end-stage renal disease continuing to increase for the foreseeable future. Already, the number of patients with type 2 diabetes entering end-stage renal disease exceeds those with type 1 diabetes.

This book is aimed principally at the multiprofessional primary care team, with the emphasis on management of patients with type 2 diabetes. However, many of the messages imparted will apply equally to patients with type 1 diabetes and renal disease.

The book has been written with two intentions in mind: to draw attention to the size of the problem of diabetic renal disease, and to demonstrate how adequate screening and early treatment can prevent or ameliorate many of the associated complications and, at the very least, slow progression of the disease. Much has been learnt in recent years about the pathogenesis, natural history and management of diabetic nephropathy.

The first chapter outlines the epidemiology of type 2 diabetes and discusses its long-term vascular complications, with particular emphasis on diabetic nephropathy. It is followed by a chapter on the pathogenesis and history of diabetic renal disease. The evidence base underlying current prevention and treatment strategies is reviewed in the third chapter, with the focus on multiple cardiovascular risk factor intervention. This includes, most importantly, control of hypertension, but also addresses dyslipidaemia and glycaemia.

There is now a large body of evidence supporting the role of newer agents that inhibit the renin angiotensin system (ACE inhibitors and angiotensin II receptor blockers) in both preventing the development of diabetic renal disease and limiting its progression, and these agents form the subject of the fourth chapter. Evidence from clinical trials suggests that they can provide a level of cardiac and renal protection greater than can be achieved through lowering of the blood pressure alone, and they are an essential part of modern diabetes management.

The penultimate chapter considers risk reduction in more detail and offers some practical advice on screening for diabetic nephropathy, assessing risk in individual patients, and identifying and treating risk factors. The final chapter concludes with a brief look at multi-professional management and the organisation of care.

I hope that readers will find this book to be an informative and practical guide to one of the most serious complications of diabetes.

A.H. Barnett

DIABETES

renal disease

A.H. BARNETT

Professor of Medicine, University of Birmingham,
and Consultant Physician, Birmingham Heartlands
and Solihull NHS Trust (Teaching)

Medical Education Partnership Ltd

Contents

1 Epidemiology and vascular complications

Type 2 diabetes is one of the great health issues of our time. The disease has reached epidemic proportions in both developed and developing countries, and the World Health Organization (WHO) has equated the public health consequences of diabetes to those of cigarette smoking[1].

Epidemiology of type 2 diabetes

The number of patients with type 2 diabetes stands at around 200 million worldwide, and it has been estimated that this will rise to 366 million within the next 25 years[1,2]. Diabetes UK reports that there are about 1.5 million people with the condition in the UK, with a further million undiagnosed, and predicts that the number of individuals diagnosed with type 2 diabetes will approach 3 million within the next few years (Fig 1.1). Predictions in the US, where the problem is even greater, suggest that a child born there today has a one-in-three chance of developing type 2 diabetes during his or her lifetime.

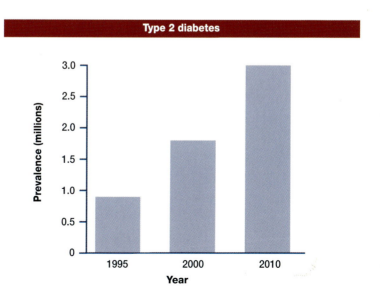

Fig 1.1 Increasing prevalence rates of (mainly type 2) diabetes in the UK – projected to the year 2010 (adapted with permission from *Diabet Med* 1997; 14 [Suppl 5]: 57-85).

The role of obesity

A major underlying cause of the increase in type 2 diabetes is obesity, which is now occurring in epidemic proportions in both developed and developing nations[3,4]. Obesity itself has important consequences for health: other than the greatly increased risk of type 2 diabetes, it is associated with cardiovascular disease, certain types of malignancy, arthritis, and psychological and other health problems. Obesity is the major driver of the epidemic of type 2 diabetes[5] and, indeed, a combination of obesity and family history accounts for around 90% of the aetiological load in type 2 diabetes (Fig 1.2). The main reason for the increase in obesity rates is thought to be diet, and it is true that many populations now consume food that is much too high in fat and sugar. The important point, though, is that our bodies can no longer cope with such diets because of reductions in physical activity. Activity levels have plummeted in many countries, including the UK, over the past two to three decades[6]. We tend to ride around in cars, sit at desks/in front of computer screens all day and then watch television or sit in the pub in the evening. Many people take little or no exercise and, in an environment where food is plentiful, there is little need to push ourselves. It is not surprising, therefore, that as a nation we are becoming increasingly obese!

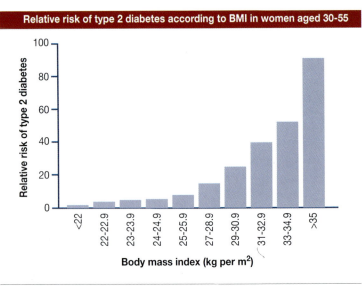

Fig 1.2 Increased risk of type 2 diabetes in association with increasing BMI (adapted from Colditz et al, 1995[5]).

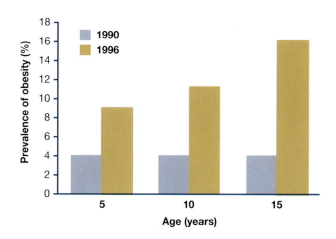

Prevalence of obesity in English children

Fig 1.3 Prevalence of obesity (body mass index >95th percentile) in nationally representative samples of English children in 1990 and 1996. The figures are even worse now! (Adapted from Reilly and Dorosty, *Lancet* 1999[7] with permission from Elsevier.)

The problem is in many ways even more serious in the child population, for similar reasons[7] (Fig 1.3). Around 15–20% of teenagers are now clinically obese and over one-third are overweight. Again, the easy availability of 'junk' food, highly processed and containing large proportions of fat and sugar, together with inadequate time and little or no encouragement to exercise, is fuelling the obesity epidemic. Vending machines dispensing chocolate bars and high-sugar drinks are ubiquitous in schools, where they generate profit. Misinformation and mislabelling of foods is common across the board. Organised sports may even be discouraged in some schools, and successive governments have allowed school playing fields to be sold off.

In the UK, the consequence is that obesity rates in adults trebled or even quadrupled, from around 6% to 20% in men and 22% in women between 1980 and 1997[3] (Fig 1.4). Overall, around 65% of the UK population are either obese or overweight, and the problem is getting worse. At the present rate of increase, obesity in the UK will overtake that in the US in around 20 years!

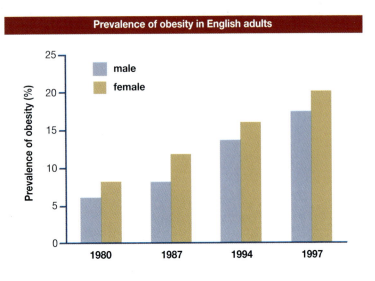

Fig 1.4 Trebling of obesity rates in English adults between 1980 and 1997 (data from the Office of Population Censuses and Surveys, and Health Surveys for England, cited in: *Obesity: Report of the British Nutrition Foundation Task Force.* Blackwell Scientific, 1999. Figure adapted with permission from *Obesity in Practice* 1999; 1(1): 2–3).

Vascular complications of diabetes

Diabetes brings a number of long-term health consequences. The vascular complications of type 2 diabetes can be summarised as follows:

- *Microangiopathy (small vessel disease)* This disease category includes diabetic retinopathy, which is the most frequent cause of blindness in the working population in the UK (Figs 1.5–1.10), as well as diabetic renal disease (nephropathy). The latter is itself associated with greatly increased cardiovascular morbidity and mortality and is also the most common cause of chronic renal failure and need for dialysis in the UK and many other countries[8,9] (Fig 1.11).
- *Large vessel (macrovascular) disease* Around 80% of patients with diabetes will die, many prematurely, from cardiovascular disease, including coronary heart disease, stroke and peripheral vascular disease[10–13] (Figs 1.12–1.15).
- *Diabetic neuropathy* This condition is thought to be caused by a combination of microvascular and metabolic abnormalities. Diabetic neuropathy will not be considered further in this book.

Fig 1.5 Diabetic background retinopathy with microaneurysms, blot haemorrhages and hard exudates.

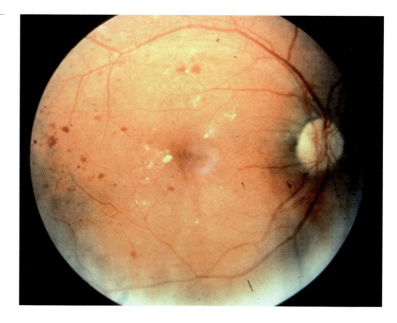

Fig 1.6 Hard exudates coalescing around the macula region of the eye (indicative of maculopathy, which can cause blindness).

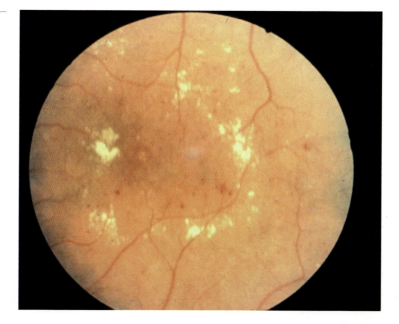

Fig 1.7
Preproliferative
retinopathy with soft
exudates and vascular
dilation.

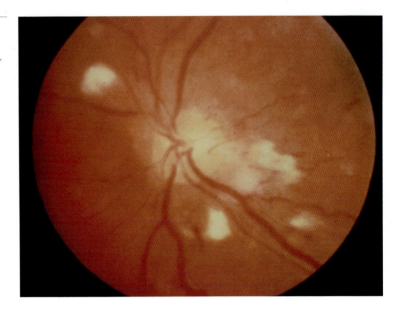

Fig 1.8 New vessels
(proliferative
retinopathy) over the
optic disc growing into
the vitreous.

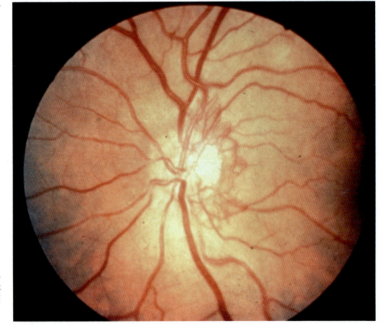

Fig 1.9 End-stage retinopathy with massive vitreous haemorrhage, fibrosis and retinal detachment. The eye is blind.

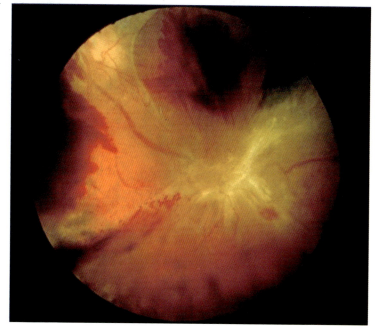

Fig 1.10 New vessels in the anterior chamber of the eye, which can lead to glaucoma and blindness.

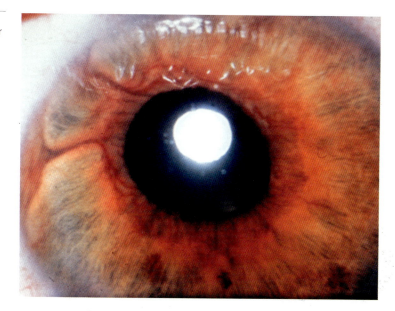

Fig 1.11 Increase in number of patients with diabetes going into end-stage renal disease in Europe over a 20-year period (adapted with permission from Raine, AEG. *Diabetologia* 1993; 36: 1099-104).

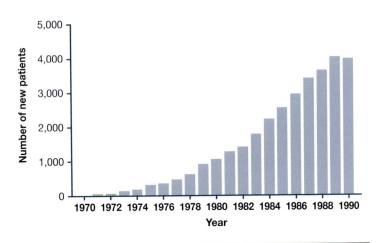

Incidence of end-stage renal disease due to diabetes in Europe

Fig 1.12 Myocardial infarction in man with type 2 diabetes – post-mortem specimen.

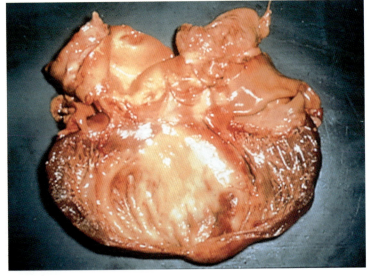

Epidemiology of diabetic renal disease

For years, renal disease was readily recognised as a complication of type 1 diabetes, with reported prevalence rates ranging from 25–40%[14]. It was identified by a characteristic combination of type 1 diabetes and persistent proteinuria, normally in association with hypertension, with progressive deterioration of renal function over time, leading eventually to death from uraemia or cardiovascular

Fig 1.13 Stroke in person with type 2 diabetes – post-mortem specimen.

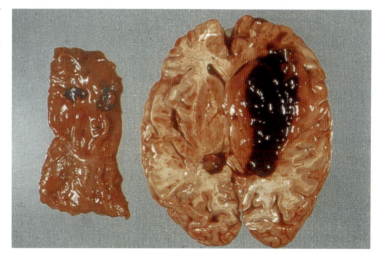

Fig 1.14 Consequence of peripheral vascular disease.

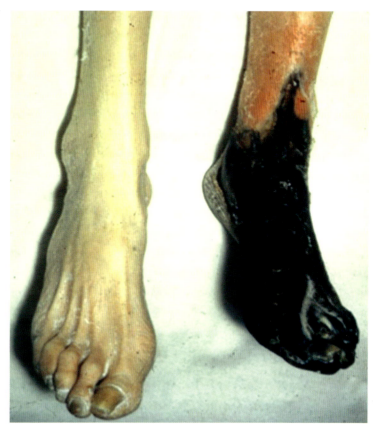

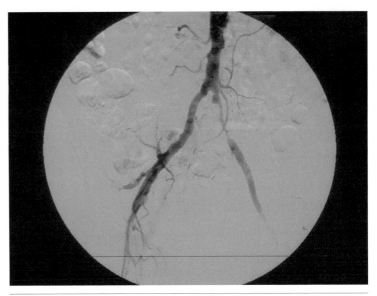

Fig 1.15 Angiogram showing arterial narrowing in peripheral vasculature consequent on peripheral vascular disease (courtesy of Dr J Henderson).

disease. With the advent of improved therapies for blood pressure control, particularly inhibitors of the renin angiotensin system, the prevalence of this complication has been reduced, although individuals with type 1 diabetes still have a risk of renal disease of around 20–25%. The stages of diabetic nephropathy have been well delineated in type 1 diabetes (Fig 1.16), but less so in type 2 diabetes.

Renal disease in type 2 diabetes has largely been overlooked by non-specialists, mainly because so many patients die from cardiovascular disease long before they develop uraemia[15]. However, it is now known that between one-quarter and one-third of patients with type 2 diabetes show evidence of renal disease, defined as persistent proteinuria in association with hypertension[16].

In recent years it has become possible to screen for the earlier phases of diabetic renal disease (incipient nephropathy) by measuring albumin excretion rate (AER) to determine the presence of microalbuminuria, defined as an AER above the normal range but below the level of 'dipstick' detection. Microalbuminuria is a strong predictor of later development of overt diabetic nephropathy and is itself associated with a greatly increased risk of morbidity and mortality from cardiovascular disease. A number of studies have suggested that microalbuminuria may be present in up to 40% of

Fig 1.16 Natural history of nephropathy in type 1 diabetes.

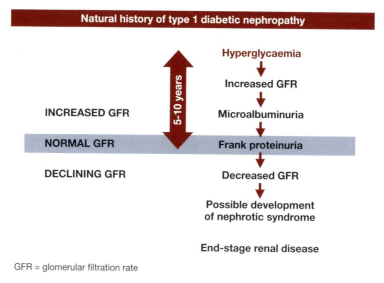

patients with type 2 diabetes[17-19]. Both microalbuminuria and overt macroproteinuria are commonly seen even at diagnosis of diabetes, testifying to the fact that a large proportion of these patients will have had some degree of glucose intolerance for many years. It is not surprising, therefore, that around one-half of all patients newly diagnosed with type 2 diabetes show some evidence of long-term vascular complications, particularly cardiovascular disease[20].

Fig 1.17 Doubling of mortality in patients with microalbuminuria compared with those with normoalbuminuria over a 10-year period (adapted with permission from Jarrett RJ et al, *Diabet Med* 1984[23]).

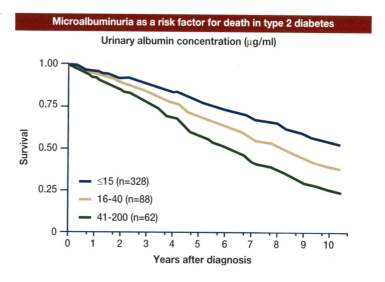

A finding of microalbuminuria in a patient with type 2 diabetes is significant: around 5% of these individuals go on to develop overt diabetic nephropathy every year[21,22]. Furthermore, renal protein leakage, even at this level, is associated with a doubling or even trebling of mortality[23–27]. Indeed, epidemiological data suggest that a patient with type 2 diabetes who is normoalbuminuric has a 40% chance of dying over a 10-year period, compared with an 80% chance in the same individual with microalbuminuria[23] (Fig 1.17). As early as five years after diagnosis of microalbuminuria, around 35% of patients have died. This figure rises to 50% in those with overt proteinuria.

The consequences of diabetic nephropathy include the need for dialysis. In the UK, around one-quarter of those undergoing dialysis have diabetes; in the US, the proportion is 40–50%[26]. The cost of dialysis for patients with diabetes in the UK now amounts to over £300 million per year. This does not include additional indirect costs to the patients, their families and society, and in no way allows for the devastating effects on quality of life seen in this group of patients.

KEY LEARNING POINTS

There are currently 1.5 million people diagnosed with diabetes in the UK, and this number is expected to double within the next few years, largely owing to the increased prevalence of obesity

Diabetic renal disease (nephropathy) will affect between one-quarter and one-third of those with type 2 diabetes

If not adequately managed, diabetic renal disease leads to significant increases in cardiovascular morbidity and mortality

Diabetic nephropathy is the most common single reason for chronic renal failure and need for dialysis in many countries in western Europe and the US

---

2 Pathogenesis and natural history

As noted in Chapter 1, changes in kidney function have been observed in patients at the time they are first diagnosed with type 2 diabetes, indicating that one or more of the major risk factors for diabetic renal disease – duration of diabetes, hypertension and other metabolic disturbances, cigarette smoking and protein overload – have been present for some time prior to diagnosis.

Pathogenesis

The histological hallmark of diabetic nephropathy is diabetic glomerulosclerosis (Figs 2.1 and 2.2). It is the result of a haemodynamic state in which glomerular filtration rate is decreased. A number of metabolic factors are also involved[27]:

- glycation of long-lived tissue proteins, including collagen
- increase in various growth factors involved in collagen synthesis
- reduction in negatively charged proteoglycans and sialic acid, resulting in loss of permselectivity within the glomerulus.

The basic lesion in the microvascular process is capillary basement membrane thickening with increased leakiness (Figs 2.3 and 2.4), which leads to the development of advanced glycation endproducts where glucose chemically attaches to long-lived tissue protein such as collagen. This is a generalised process and leakiness of plasma protein in one vascular bed often indicates similar abnormalities elsewhere. This may explain why microalbuminuria is not just a risk factor for later development of chronic renal failure, but also points to 'leaky' or 'bad' blood vessels elsewhere in the body, including other parts of the cardiovascular system.

Natural history

Functional changes within the kidney may soon be followed by structural changes (Fig 2.5). The latter include glomerular basement membrane thickening, mesangial expansion and other microvascular changes. More than one-half of patients are hypertensive at diagnosis of type 2 diabetes. This problem progresses with time such that around 80% of patients with type 2 diabetes will develop hypertension, including almost all of those with proteinuria[28, 29]. At diagnosis, around one-fifth of patients with

Fig 2.1 Haemotoxylin and eosin stain showing glomerulus with normal histological architecture.

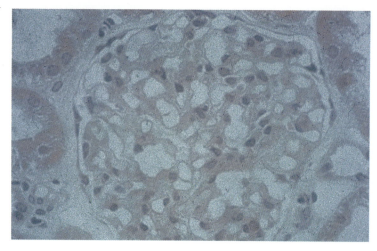

Fig 2.2 Haemotoxylin and eosin stain showing loss of normal histological architecture and basement membrane thickening in a patient with type 2 diabetes, hypertension and proteinuria.

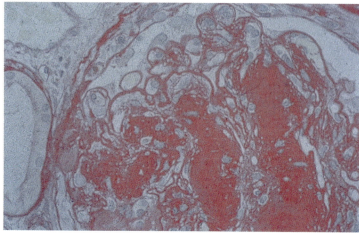

type 2 diabetes are already microalbuminuric and this proportion may rise to 30–40% over time[17–19]. Microalbuminuria heralds the later development of overt proteinuria, although, again, a percentage of newly diagnosed patients with type 2 diabetes will already have overt macroproteinuria at diagnosis. Without intervention, microalbuminuria will convert to overt proteinuria in around 5–10% of these patients each year[17–19]. Overt, persistent macroproteinuria is followed by a rise in serum creatinine levels and again, without intervention, end-stage renal disease will eventually develop, unless the patient dies before this stage is reached.

Fig 2.3 Electron micrograph of healthy capillary in cross-section, showing normal basement membrane thickness.

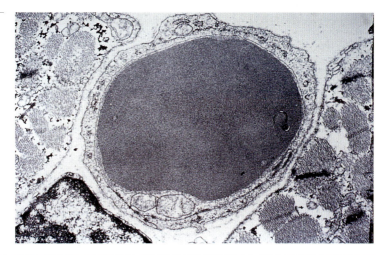

Fig 2.4 Electron micrograph of capillary from patient with longstanding diabetes showing basement membrane thickening and leakiness – histological hallmarks of microangiopathy.

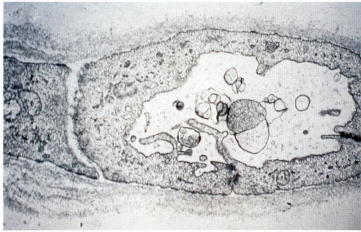

Overarching this sequence is a massively increased risk of cardiovascular morbidity and mortality. Indeed, hypertension and proteinuria in a patient with type 2 diabetes is a most ominous finding, with an extremely poor prognosis unless effective interventions are instituted.

However, it is important to note that microalbuminuria alone is associated with a doubling of mortality in type 2 diabetes. Without intervention, around 80% of such patients would be expected to die, usually from cardiovascular disease, within 10 years of diagnosis[23]. This is twice the mortality rate expected in normo-albuminuric patients.

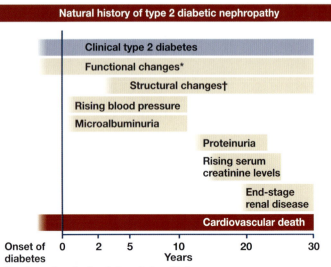

Natural history of type 2 diabetic nephropathy

| Clinical type 2 diabetes |
| Functional changes* |
| Structural changes† |
| Rising blood pressure |
| Microalbuminuria |
| Proteinuria |
| Rising serum creatinine levels |
| End-stage renal disease |
| Cardiovascular death |

Onset of diabetes: 0 2 5 10 20 30
Years

*Renal haemodynamics altered, glomerular hyperfiltration
† Glomerular basement membrane thickening↑, mesangial expansion↑, microvascular changes +/-

Fig 2.5 Natural history of renal disease in type 2 diabetes. Abnormalities may be detected even at diagnosis of diabetes and, without intervention, will progress to end-stage renal disease or cardiovascular death.

The situation is even worse for patients with overt proteinuria: 50% of these individuals will die within five years of diagnosis, usually from cardiovascular disease.

Disease stages

Although the natural history of nephropathy in type 1 diabetes has been well described, this is not the case in renal disease associated with type 2 diabetes. Clinically, nephropathy in type 2 diabetes is recognised on the basis of either micro- or macroalbuminuria, normally in association with hypertension, which, without intervention, will lead to a progressive decline in renal function and a massively increased risk of cardiovascular death.

For practical purposes, nephropathy in type 2 diabetes is usually divided into two stages:
- *Incipient nephropathy* This refers to the phase of microalbuminuria that is confirmed on the basis of a urinary albumin excretion rate of 20–200µg/min. As discussed above, even this small but increased protein leakage is associated with serious morbidity and mortality. At this stage the process may

be reversed or at least stabilised (see later chapters). It is therefore important for physicians to screen for microalbuminuria and, if present, actively intervene at this stage in the disease process.

● *Overt nephropathy* A finding of persistent dipstick-positive proteinuria in a person with type 2 diabetes, almost always in association with hypertension, and in the absence of other causes such as urinary tract infection, indicates overt nephropathy. This is an extremely ominous finding and, as previously discussed, is associated with massively increased cardiovascular morbidity and mortality and later development of end-stage renal disease, if the patient survives long enough. Progression to frank renal failure can be slowed or even stabilised at this stage, but cannot be reversed with current treatment methods. Overt proteinuria with leakage beyond 200µg/min tends to increase with time and is commonly associated (as is microalbuminuria) with a range of other cardiovascular risk factors, particularly dyslipidaemia and hypertension. These patients need extremely aggressive blood pressure management, together with other therapies aimed at cardiovascular protection.

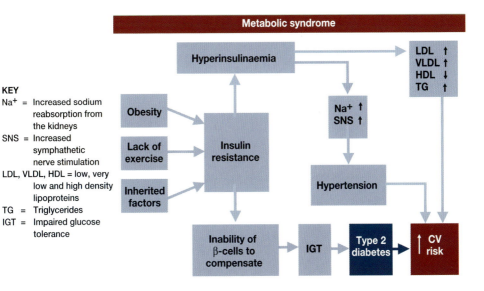

KEY
Na⁺ = Increased sodium reabsorption from the kidneys
SNS = Increased sympathetic nerve stimulation
LDL, VLDL, HDL = low, very low and high density lipoproteins
TG = Triglycerides
IGT = Impaired glucose tolerance

Fig 2.6 Schematic diagram of the metabolic syndrome (syndrome of chronic cardiovascular risk) showing the association of insulin resistance with a range of cardiovascular risk factors.

Proteinuria and other cardiovascular risk factors

The very strong association between diabetic nephropathy, even during the incipient phase, and cardiovascular death is both remarkable and frightening! It is in part explained by the fact that leakiness of blood vessels in the kidney is a marker for generalised problems elsewhere within the vasculature, including the coronary and cerebral arteries. Beyond this, patients with nephropathy are almost always hypertensive and many suffer from dyslipidaemia. Indeed, micro- or macroalbuminuria has been included in some definitions of the metabolic syndrome (syndrome of chronic cardiovascular risk), which is so prevalent in patients with diabetes[30] (Fig 2.6). The classic dyslipidaemia of metabolic syndrome consists of low levels of high-density lipoproteins (HDL), raised triglycerides and an increase in small, dense low-density lipoproteins (LDL) – a highly atherogenic profile. The mechanism underlying these associations, which may include insulin resistance as a central feature, will not be discussed further in this book.

Finally, it is important to emphasise that not only should type 2 diabetes be viewed as a cardiovascular disease, but that the presence of nephropathy, commonly associated with other cardiovascular risk factors, heralds a particularly aggressive form of arteriosclerosis with extremely poor prognosis unless optimal intervention occurs. This intervention should take place as early as possible in the disease process.

KEY LEARNING POINTS

Changes in kidney function have been observed in patients at the time of diagnosis of diabetes, indicating the presence of risk factors for some time prior to diagnosis

Functional changes may soon be followed by structural changes

Around 80% of patients with type 2 diabetes will develop hypertension, including almost all of those with proteinuria

The histological hallmark of diabetic renal disease (nephropathy) is diabetic glomerulosclerosis

In type 2 diabetes, nephropathy is divided into two major stages: incipient (microalbuminuria) and overt (macroalbuminuria)

Incipient nephropathy is a strong predictor of later development of overt nephropathy and is itself associated with a greatly increased risk of cardiovascular morbidity and mortality

3 Evidence base for prevention and treatment

The major risk factors for development and progression of diabetic renal disease are degree of metabolic control and presence of hypertension. It goes without saying that diabetic renal disease only develops in the presence of diabetes! Interestingly, at least in type 1 diabetes, improving glycaemic control does not appear to stop or reverse the progression of nephropathy from the incipient to the overt stage.

There is little doubt that the most important risk factor for progression and, possibly, initiation of diabetic nephropathy is hypertension[15-19]. Hypertension *per se* is associated with raised plasma volume caused by increased exchangeable body sodium[30]. These abnormalities may precede the onset of hypertension. In addition, the renin angiotensin system (RAS) is pivotal in the maintenance of normal blood pressure through its regulation of vascular tone and sodium/water homeostasis[31]. There is now good evidence to indicate that the RAS is over-activated in diabetes, for reasons that are as yet undetermined[32].

There are also data, particularly those gleaned from animal studies, which point to raised intraglomerular pressure as a central feature of nephropathy. Again, this may be an effect of an over-activated RAS[33].

Although the exact mechanism underlying the relationship between diabetes and hypertension is unclear, we know that around 80% of patients with type 2 diabetes will be hypertensive and, of these, around one-third will go on to develop diabetic renal disease.

Evidence from clinical trials
DCCT and UKPDS

Two major studies, one in type 1 diabetes (Diabetes Control and Complications Trial – DCCT[34]) and the other in type 2 diabetes (United Kingdom Prospective Diabetes Study – UKPDS[20]), have shown conclusively that strict glycaemic control significantly reduces the incidence of nephropathy (Table 3.1). Prior to the publication of the UKPDS results in 1998, all the evidence for the benefits of blood pressure-lowering in patients with diabetes had been extrapolated from data taken from the general population.

Table 3.1: UKPDS data showing reductions in incidence of microvascular disease, including diabetic nephropathy, myocardial infarction and other diabetes-related endpoints, in patients randomised to strict compared to conventional glycaemic control[20]

Endpoint	Relative risk	p
Microvascular disease (including nephropathy)	↓ 25%	0.010
Myocardial infarction	↓ 16%	0.052
Other diabetes-related endpoints	↓ 12%	0.029

Strict glycaemic control = HbA_{1c} 7.0%
Conventional glycaemic control = HbA_{1c} 7.9%

The UKPDS showed clearly the benefits of both improved glucose control and of treatment to lower blood pressure[35] (Table 3.2). In that study, hypertensive subjects were randomised into strict and conventional blood pressure control groups and, over the nine-year study period, there emerged a clear separation of 10mmHg systolic and 5mmHg diastolic blood pressure in favour of strict control. This was associated with dramatic risk reductions in vascular endpoints and mortality and, in the context of this book, significant reductions in the incidence of nephropathy.

HOT

Since then, many trials have supported the benefits of tight blood pressure control in patients with diabetes. The Hypertension

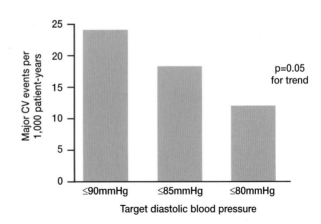

Fig 3.1 Cardiovascular event rates in subjects with diabetes were halved in the group randomised to strict blood pressure control (diastolic <80mmHg) compared with those randomised to less strict blood pressure control (diastolic <90mmHg) in the HOT trial (adapted from Hansson L, et al. *Lancet* 1998[36] with permission from Elsevier).

HOT: benefits of strict blood pressure control in patients with diabetes

p=0.05 for trend

Major CV events per 1,000 patient-years

≤90mmHg   ≤85mmHg   ≤80mmHg

Target diastolic blood pressure

Table 3.2: UKPDS data showing reductions in incidence of microvascular disease, other diabetes-related endpoints, deaths related to diabetes and stroke, in patients randomised to strict compared to conventional blood pressure control[35]

Endpoint	Relative risk	p
Microvascular disease	↓ 37%	0.010
Other diabetes-related endpoints	↓ 24%	0.005
Deaths related to diabetes	↓ 32%	0.020
Stroke	↓ 44%	0.013

Strict blood pressure control = 142/82mmHg
Conventional blood pressure control = 154/87mmHg

Optimal Treatment (HOT) study recruited 20,000 patients, including a large cohort with type 2 diabetes[36]. They were randomised into three groups, with target diastolic blood pressures of <80mmHg, <85mmHg and <90mmHg. In the subgroup with diabetes, there was a reduction of approximately 50% in major cardiovascular events in the group randomised to the lowest target blood pressure (<80mmHg) compared to those in the group with the highest target blood pressure (<90mmHg) (Fig 3.1). The HOT study also reported that treatment with low-dose aspirin (75mg daily) was associated with a reduction of approximately 15% in cardiovascular endpoints and mortality, albeit at the expense of an increased risk of non-fatal haemorrhage.

Fig 3.2 Data from the HOPE study showing reduction in the primary composite endpoint of myocardial infarction, stroke or death in subjects with diabetes treated with the ACE inhibitor ramipril (adapted from HOPE Study Investigators. *Lancet* 2000[40] with permission from Elsevier).

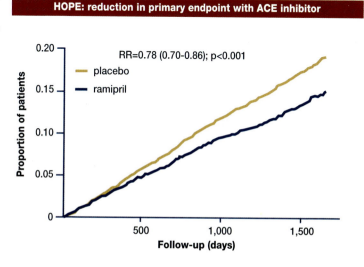

HOPE: reduction in primary endpoint with ACE inhibitor

RR=0.78 (0.70-0.86); p<0.001

placebo
ramipril

Proportion of patients

Follow-up (days)

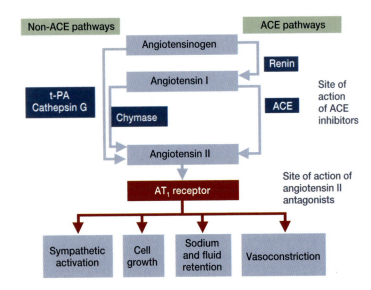

Fig 3.3 The renin angiotensin system and the sites of action of ACE inhibitors and angiotensin receptor blockers (adapted from Thompson Publishing Services. In: *Clinical Management of Hypertension*. Barnett AH [ed]. London: Martin Dunitz, 2002; 52).

Other trials

A number of other studies have also demonstrated the benefits of antihypertensive treatment in reducing cardiovascular morbidity and mortality in patients with diabetes. They include the Systolic Hypertension in the Elderly Programme (SHEP)[37], the SYSTolic Hypertension in EURope (SYST-EUR) trial[38], the CAPtopril Prevention Project (CAPPP)[39] and the Heart Outcomes Prevention Evaluation (HOPE) study[40] (Fig 3.2). All of these trials reported significant reductions in cardiovascular event rates and mortality.

The most important message from all of these clinical trials is: *Get the blood pressure down and keep it down!*

Which agents?

Trials that have specifically recruited patients with type 2 diabetes and nephropathy have tended to focus on agents that inhibit the RAS – angiotensin-converting enzyme (ACE) inhibitors and angiotensin II receptor blockers (ARBs) As discussed above, the RAS is intimately involved in the maintenance of blood pressure and the development of hypertension. ACE inhibitors work indirectly in the RAS by inhibiting angiotensin-converting enzyme, while ARBs exert a direct blocking effect on the angiotensin II receptor[41] (Fig 3.3). Both CAPPP and the HOPE study used ACE inhibitors, and both reported better

Fig 3.4 Data showing significant reduction in albumin excretion rate in favour of ACE inhibition (lisinopril) compared with calcium channel blockade (nifedipine) (adapted from Agardh CD, et al. *J Human Hypertens* 1996[43]).

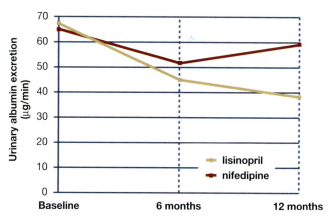

Urinary albumin excretion rates in patients treated with lisinopril and nifedipine at baseline and after 6 and 12 months. Data presented as median

outcomes with these agents than with standard antihypertensive therapies.

The HOPE investigators also made the suggestion, based on the results of their subgroup analysis, that the ACE inhibitor might have provided a degree of renal protection over and above that conferred by lowering of the blood pressure alone[40]. This finding has been echoed in several other studies that have reported reductions in proteinuria in subjects given ACE inhibitors that appear to be greater than those seen in subjects given other anti-hypertensive agents (excluding ARBs) or placebo[27]. Some early, small studies also showed a decrease in the rate of progression of microalbuminuria in subjects given a β-blocker together with a diuretic[42]. Larger studies that used ACE inhibitors include a multi-centre, double-blind, randomised, parallel-group comparison of over 300 patients with type 2 diabetes and microalbuminuria[43]. Subjects were randomised to receive either the ACE inhibitor lisinopril or the calcium channel blocker nifedipine for one year. Despite the fact that blood pressure and glucose control were similar in the two groups, there was a significant reduction in urinary albumin excretion in the lisinopril group compared with the nifedipine group (Fig 3.4).

Recent work has therefore been focused on inhibitors of the RAS, and these agents form the subject of the next chapter.

KEY LEARNING POINTS

The primary risk factors for development of nephropathy are poor metabolic control and hypertension

Hypertension is also the single most important risk factor for progression of existing nephropathy

There is good evidence showing that strict glycaemic control will reduce the incidence of nephropathy. Attention to glycaemic control in all patients with diabetes is worth while and will yield clear health benefits

Once a patient develops incipient or overt nephropathy, the best evidence base is for very tight blood pressure control. A combination of antihypertensive agents from different classes will usually be required if the patient is to get even close to target blood pressure (ideally <125/75mmHg)

4 The role of newer agents

Although a range of studies have shown reductions in microalbuminuria through inhibition of the RAS with an ACE inhibitor, most have concentrated on patients with type 1 diabetes and it is fair to say that, until recently, the strongest evidence of renal protection in terms of hard endpoints has been limited to data produced by studies of patients with type 1 diabetes and advanced nephropathy[44]. This has now changed, however, with publication of the DETAIL trial, which is discussed more comprehensively below[41].

Evidence from clinical trials
ACE inhibitors and calcium channel blockers: BENEDICT
The renoprotective properties of ACE inhibitors have been shown in the multicentre, double-blind, randomised BErgano NEphrologic DIabetes Complications Trial (BENEDICT)[45]. This study was designed to assess whether ACE inhibitors and non-dihydropyridine calcium channel blockers (CCBs), alone or in combination, would prevent microalbuminuria in subjects with hypertension, type 2 diabetes and normal urinary albumin excretion. Over 1,200 subjects were randomised to receive treatment for at least three years with the ACE inhibitor trandolapril plus the CCB verapamil; trandolapril alone; verapamil alone; or placebo. The target blood pressure was 120/80mmHg and the primary endpoint was the development of persistent microalbuminuria, defined as an overnight albumin excretion rate (AER) >20µg/min on two consecutive occasions.

The primary outcome was reached in around 6% of subjects receiving either trandolapril plus verapamil, or trandolapril alone, compared with 12% of the subjects receiving verapamil alone and 10% of those receiving placebo. Thus, trandolapril plus verapamil, and trandolapril alone, delayed the onset of microalbuminuria by 2.6 and 2.1 times respectively. The conclusion from this study is that ACE inhibition has a renoprotective effect, reducing the risk of development of incipient (and presumably also overt) nephropathy in subjects with type 2 diabetes. This benefit appears to be over and above that achieved by reduction in blood pressure alone, given that the group taking solely the CCB and the placebo group achieved similar blood pressures, but with much more rapid progression to incipient nephropathy. These results support the view that not only does inhibition of the RAS protect the already damaged kidney in type 2 diabetes, it also reduces the risk of the complication developing in the first place.

Angiotensin II receptor blockers (ARBs): LIFE and CHARM
This relatively new class of agents acts through a direct blocking effect at the angiotensin II receptor[31]. ARBs are particularly useful in the pharmacotherapy of hypertension, being:
- as efficacious as other antihypertensive agents
- metabolically neutral
- suitable for combination therapy with agents from any other antihypertensive class
- likely to be the best tolerated of all antihypertensive agents and less likely than ACE inhibitors to cause chronic cough
- known to confer both cardiac (including treatment of heart failure) and renal protection.

Cardiovascular protection was demonstrated in the Losartan Intervention For Endpoint reduction in hypertension (LIFE) trial, which compared the ARB losartan with the β-blocker atenolol in patients with left ventricular hypertrophy[46]. There was a 15% reduction (p<0.009) in the primary composite endpoint of cardiovascular mortality, fatal/non-fatal stroke or fatal/non-fatal myocardial infarction in the ARB group compared with the β-blocker group.

Beneficial effects on the heart have also been demonstrated in the Candesartan in Heart failure Assessment of Reduction in Mortality and morbidity (CHARM) programme (Fig 4.1)[47-51]. In this study, the ARB candesartan was compared with placebo in three different populations with heart failure graded NYHA Class II–IV. Three studies were carried out:
- CHARM–added, which randomised approximately 2,500 patients with ejection fractions <40% who were treated with optimum doses of ACE inhibitors
- CHARM–alternative, which randomised around 2,000 patients with ejection fractions <40% who were intolerant of ACE inhibitors
- CHARM–preserved, which randomised about 3,000 patients with ejection fractions >40%.

When the trials were combined for analysis into the CHARM–overall programme, statistically significant reductions

Fig 4.1 Effect of angiotensin receptor II blockade with candesartan on cardiovascular mortality or hospital admission for congestive heart failure in the CHARM study (adapted from Pfeffer MA, et al. *Lancet* 2003[47] with permission from Elsevier).

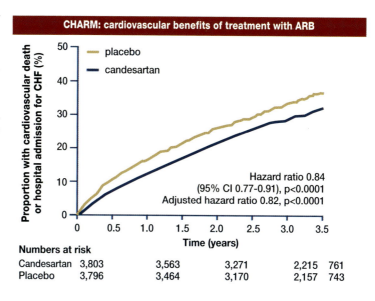

CHARM: cardiovascular benefits of treatment with ARB

Hazard ratio 0.84
(95% CI 0.77-0.91), p<0.0001
Adjusted hazard ratio 0.82, p<0.0001

Numbers at risk					
Candesartan	3,803	3,563	3,271	2,215	761
Placebo	3,796	3,464	3,170	2,157	743

were shown in the primary endpoint of mortality (10%). In addition, there was a highly significant absolute reduction in the combined incidence of cardiovascular death and hospitalisation for heart failure (16%), and a reduction in the number of patients developing diabetes of 6% versus 7.4% in the groups given candesartan. The authors concluded that ARBs should be prescribed in addition to ACE inhibitors, β-blockers and/or spironolactone in patients with ejection fractions <40%, and as an alternative to ACE inhibitors in patients with intolerance to these drugs. ARBs can also be used in patients with ejection fractions >40% to reduce the risk of hospitalisation with heart failure.

The most dramatic results of studies with ARBs, however, have been in the context of renal protection in type 2 diabetes. A number of major studies have been published in recent years, all supporting the renoprotective properties of ARBs at different stages of the disease process. These are considered in turn.

ARBs in the prevention of progression from incipient to overt nephropathy: IRMA2

The IRMA2 (IRbesartan MicroAlbuminuria in type 2 diabetic subjects) study involved almost 600 patients with type 2 diabetes, hypertension and microalbuminuria who were randomised to receive either a low dose (150mg daily) or a high dose (300mg daily) of the ARB irbesartan, or placebo[52]. The subjects were followed for two years and during that time they could receive any other antihypertensive agent (except an ACE inhibitor). The blood pressure target was the same in all three groups and, indeed, the achieved blood pressure was almost identical in the three groups. The primary endpoint was time to onset of overt nephropathy, defined as AER >200µg/min and an increase of at least 30% from baseline.

Over the duration of the study, the relative risk reductions in the treatment groups compared with the placebo group were 70% (p<0.001) in the group given high-dose irbesartan and 40% (p=0.08) in those given the lower dose (Fig 4.2). Using a 'numbers needed to treat' analysis, it was calculated that giving irbesartan 300mg daily to 10 patients for two years would prevent the progression of microalbuminuria to overt diabetic nephropathy in one patient; in other words, would be highly cost effective.

ARBs in the management of overt nephropathy in type 2 diabetes: IDNT and RENAAL

The three-year IDNT (Irbesartan in Diabetic Nephropathy Trial) recruited approximately 1,700 subjects with type 2 diabetes and hypertension. It set out to compare the effects of the ARB

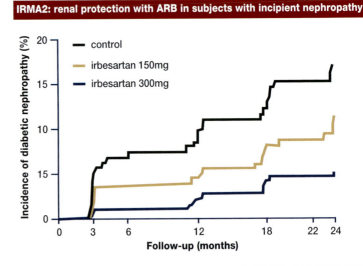

IRMA2: renal protection with ARB in subjects with incipient nephropathy

Fig 4.2 Slowing/prevention of incipient to overt nephropathy with the angiotensin receptor II blocker irbesartan in the IRMA2 study (adapted from Parving H-H, et al. *N Engl J Med* 2001[52] with permission from the Massachusetts Medical Society).

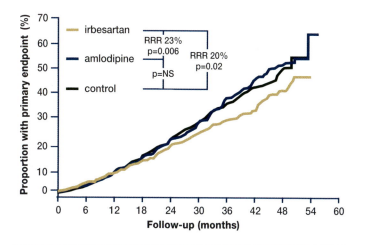

Fig 4.3 Slowing of progression of established nephropathy (primary endpoint: composite of doubling of baseline creatinine level, end-stage renal disease, and death) in IDNT study with the angiotensin receptor II blocker irbesartan (adapted from Lewis EJ, et al. *N Engl J Med* 2001[53] with permission from the Massachusetts Medical Society).

irbesartan with placebo and with the CCB amlodipine[53]. Blood pressure targets were similar in the three groups and, as in IRMA2, any other antihypertensive agent, with the exception of ACE inhibitors, could be added in all three groups. At randomisation, subjects had persistent proteinuria and either normal or raised creatinine. The primary outcome was time to a composite of doubling of baseline creatinine, end-stage renal disease and death. Irbesartan was associated with a relative risk reduction of 20% compared to placebo (p=0.02) and 23% compared to amlodipine (p=0.006) (Fig 4.3). It can be estimated that treatment of 15 hypertensive patients with significant proteinuria for three years with irbesartan would save one patient from a doubling of baseline creatinine, development of end-stage renal disease or death – again, highly cost effective!

The RENAAL (Reduction in Endpoints in patients with Non-insulin-dependent diabetes mellitus with the Angiotensin II Antagonist Losartan) study compared a different ARB, losartan, with placebo in a similar group of patients[54]. The relative risk reduction for the primary composite endpoint, which was virtually the same as that in IDNT, was 16% (p=0.02) in the treatment group compared with the control group.

Renoprotection with ARBs compared to ACE inhibitors: DETAIL

Although ACE inhibitors have been shown to confer renoprotection in patients with type 1 diabetes, in those with type 2 disease, current evidence favours the use of ARBs. There has, therefore, been much interest in head-to-head comparisons of these two types of agents and whether their use in combination would provide greater protection.

Until recently, there had been only one clinical study that directly compared the effect of an ARB (losartan) with that of an ACE inhibitor (enalapril) in subjects with type 2 diabetes and early nephropathy[55]. This study lasted only one year and found no significant difference between the two drugs; both reduced urinary albumin excretion. Three other studies that compared the two agents – two in patients who had had a myocardial infarction[56, 57] and one in subjects who had suffered heart failure[58] – did not include renal outcomes, and were not specifically focused on type 2 diabetes.

Importantly, however, we now have data from a long-term, head-to-head comparison of an ACE inhibitor with an ARB in patients with type 2 diabetes and early nephropathy[41]. The DETAIL (Diabetics Exposed to Telmisartan And enaIaprIL) study was a prospective, multicentre, double-blind, five-year investigation of 250 subjects with type 2 diabetes and early nephropathy in which the author was principal investigator. Of the subjects

Fig 4.4 Design of the Diabetics Exposed to Telmisartan And enalaprIL (DETAIL) trial (adapted from Barnett AH, et al. *N Engl J Med* 2004[41] with permission from the Massachusetts Medical Society).

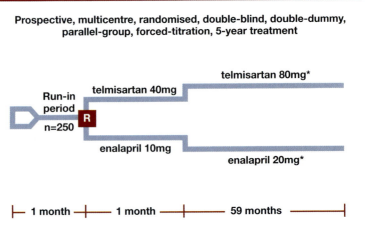

DETAIL: study design

Prospective, multicentre, randomised, double-blind, double-dummy, parallel-group, forced-titration, 5-year treatment

telmisartan 80mg*

telmisartan 40mg

Run-in period
R
n=250

enalapril 10mg

enalapril 20mg*

|— 1 month —|— 1 month —|— 59 months —|

*Optional dose reduction to telmisartan 40mg or enalapril 10mg after 2 months

Table 4.1: Data from DETAIL study showing stabilisation of renal function

Endpoint	Telmisartan group (n = 120)	Enalapril group (n = 130)	Difference	p
Mean serum creatinine (μmol/l)	+8.84	+8.84	0.00	NSD
Mean albumin excretion rate (μg/min)	-1.67	-0.33	1.34	NSD*

NSD = non-significant difference
*Determined from the logarithm of the individual change from baseline

recruited to the trial, 80% had microalbuminuria and 20% were overtly proteinuric, albeit in the earlier phases. They were randomised to receive either the ARB telmisartan or the ACE inhibitor enalapril (Fig 4.4). The primary endpoint was change in glomerular filtration rate (GFR) as measured by plasma clearance of iohexol – the 'gold standard' for assessing renal function. Secondary endpoints included annual change in GFR, serum creatinine level, urinary albumin excretion, blood pressure, rates of end-stage renal disease, and cardiovascular events and mortality.

After five years, the change in GFR was similar in the two groups, indicating equivalent renal protection (Fig 4.5). There were also no significant differences in the secondary endpoints (Table 4.1).

This study yielded a number of very important findings. There was almost complete stabilisation of renal function in both groups of subjects over the five-year study. There was an initial (and expected) fairly steep fall in GFR in the first year of the study, less so in the second year, and stabilisation beyond this time period. Indeed, for those who completed the study, the mean fall in GFR over years three, four and five and was only 2ml/min/year – not significantly different from that expected in association with ageing in the general population. The result was that not one patient in either group went into end-stage renal disease and none required dialysis. Indeed, no patient had a rise in serum creatinine beyond 200μmol/l over the five-year study period.

It is notable that in this high-risk group of subjects a mortality rate of around 35% was expected, principally from cardiovascular events. In fact, total mortality in each group was only 5%, and only one-half of this was due to a cardiovascular event (Table 4.1). This is a remarkable finding (particularly since around one-half of the patients had a history of cardiovascular disease at randomisation) and, although there was increased usage of statins, aspirin and other antihypertensive agents during the course of the study, it is

Fig 4.5 Change in glomerular filtration rate from baseline over five years and yearly in the DETAIL study. Note the almost complete stabilisation of renal function in both the ACE inhibitor (enalapril) and the angiotensin receptor II blocker (telmisartan) groups beyond three years, with no significant difference between the groups (adapted from Barnett AH, et al. *N Engl J Med* 2004[41] with permission from the Massachusetts Medical Society).

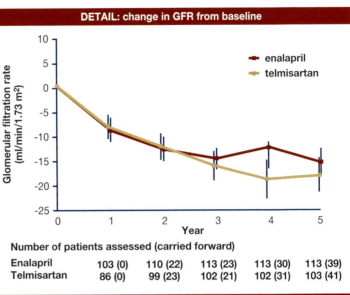

DETAIL: change in GFR from baseline

Number of patients assessed (carried forward)

	Baseline to Year 1	Year 1 to Year 2	Year 2 to Year 3	Year 3 to Year 4	Year 4 to Year 5
Enalapril	103 (0)	110 (22)	113 (23)	113 (30)	113 (39)
Telmisartan	86 (0)	99 (23)	102 (21)	102 (31)	103 (41)

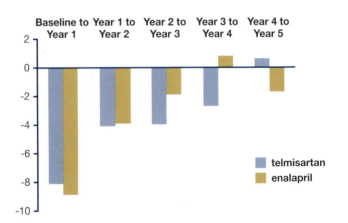

DETAIL: yearly changes in GFR

unlikely that these agents alone could account for the dramatic reduction in expected mortality rates. The assumption is that, through inhibition of the RAS, both classes of drugs conferred not just renoprotective, but also cardioprotective effects. These results support those of other studies such as HOPE, which also demonstrated profound risk reductions in cardiovascular events and mortality in higher-risk subjects, including those with diabetes, who were given an ACE inhibitor[40].

Combination of ACE inhibitors and ARBs

No long-term studies have been carried out to determine whether a combination of two different methods of inhibiting the RAS, using an ACE inhibitor combined with an ARB, would confer extra renoprotection over and above that which could be achieved using a single agent. So far, only one study using such a combination has been reported in the context of renal disease in subjects with type 2 diabetes. The results suggested that there was an additive effect in lowering blood pressure and greater reduction of proteinuria[59].

Implications for practice

The evidence we have suggests that there is a specific role for both ACE inhibitors and ARBs in renoprotection. One of these agents should be used as first-line treatment in patients with diabetic nephropathy, following these principles:

- Since the best renal protection is achieved using higher doses of ACE inhibitors and ARBs, treatment should be initiated using a low dose, but titrated up fairly rapidly to the evidence-based (normally highest) dose.
- Electrolytes should be measured 7–10 days after starting treatment with an ACE inhibitor or an ARB, and after each dose increase, in order to identify the very rare (but serious) renal deterioration that can occur when using these agents in patients with renal artery stenosis.

Table 4.2: Data from the DETAIL study showing morbidity/mortality rates. No patient developed advanced renal disease. Mortality was extremely low at 5%, compared to an expected mortality, without intervention, of 35% in this patient group

Endpoint	Telmisartan group (n = 120)	Enalapril group (n = 130)	p
End-stage renal disease [n (%)]	0 (0)	0 (0)	NSD
Cerebrovascular accident	6 (5.0)	6 (4.6)	NSD
Congestive heart failure	9 (7.5)	7 (5.4)	NSD
Non-fatal myocardial infarction	9 (7.5)	6 (4.6)	NSD
Deaths	6 (5.0)	6 (4.6)	NSD
Cardiovascular deaths	3 (2.5)	2 (1.5)	NSD

NSD = non-significant difference

- Although an ACE inhibitor or an ARB should be the first-line antihypertensive treatment in patients with diabetic nephropathy, drugs from any other class of antihypertensive agent can be added to help reduce blood pressure to the target level. The author's usual first-line combination is an inhibitor of the RAS together with a thiazide or thiazide-like diuretic.
- Given the fact that 80% of patients with type 2 diabetes are hypertensive, and the increasing evidence showing vascular protection with ACE inhibitors and ARBs, one of these agents should normally be used in the management of hypertension, even in patients who show no evidence of nephropathy.

KEY LEARNING POINTS

There is now a very good evidence base showing that agents which inhibit the renin angiotensin sysem – ACE inhibitors and angiotensin II receptor blockers (ARBs) – have reno- and cardioprotective properties over and above those expected from simply lowering blood pressure

An ACE inhibitor or an ARB should be the usual first-line treatment in the management of both incipient and overt diabetic nephropathy

There is also a good rationale supporting the use of these agents as first-line treatment in the management of hypertension in diabetes generally

5 Risk reduction: an overview

Although diabetic renal disease is a grave complication, this is an area of medicine where profound health benefit can be achieved with correct management. Practitioners need to appreciate how common diabetic nephropathy is, and must try to identify the problem as early as possible, preferably at the incipient stage. This is because, with the right management, progression to overt nephropathy may be prevented or at least dramatically retarded.

Screening for hypertension and micro- and macroalbuminuria is a vital part of such management. If present, these conditions need to be treated aggressively to prevent both further progression of renal disease and an increase in the risk of cardiovascular events and mortality.

Screening

The earlier nephropathy can be picked up, the better the long-term outlook[41, 45, 52]. Even at the microalbuminuric stage, risk is considerably increased and intervention is vital. Around 30–40% of patients with type 2 diabetes may have microalbuminuria and, indeed, even at diagnosis significant numbers have this complication. For these reasons, screening for microalbuminuria and identification of overt proteinuria are important parts of management in type 2 diabetes.

There are simple, semi-quantitative dipstick tests for microalbuminuria which, if positive, should generate a laboratory assessment. Although measurement of 24-hour or overnight albumin excretion is the 'gold standard', it is much simpler, and equally good, to take a spot urine and ask the laboratory for measurement of an albumin:creatinine ratio (ACR). The reference ranges are different in men and women (≥ 2.5mg/mmol and ≥ 3.5mg/mmol respectively). If the ACR is raised on two or more occasions and there are no other causes, such as a urinary tract infection, then a diagnosis of incipient nephropathy can be made. Particular attention must then be paid to cardiovascular risk factors (see below) and specific plans made to limit kidney damage.

Identification of either micro- or macroproteinuria, almost always in association with hypertension, should generate a number of other investigations, if these have not recently been done:

- measurement of electrolytes and, where available (now in many laboratories), an estimated glomerular filtration rate (GFRe)
- full blood count in patients with raised creatinine or reduced GFR, as many will be anaemic
- lipid profile (ideally total cholesterol, LDL and HDL cholesterol and, possibly, triglycerides)
- ECG
- normally a renal ultrasound, although in many hospitals the waiting list for this investigation is extremely long.

Overt, dipstick-positive macroproteinuria, indicating disease progression, is an ominous finding. A combination of type 2 diabetes, hypertension and overt proteinuria denotes an extremely poor prognosis unless rapid and aggressive intervention is carried out. The two important areas for major consideration are cardiac and renal protection.

Managing risk factors
Hypertension

The vast majority of these patients will be hypertensive and even for the few who are normotensive it is still wise to start treatment with an inhibitor of the RAS. This should be either an ACE inhibitor or an ARB.

No limit has yet been determined below which further renal benefit cannot be achieved by blood pressure lowering. The most recent guidelines issued by the British Hypertension Society for the management of hypertension in diabetes have suggested a target blood pressure of <130/80mmHg (audit standard <140/80mmHg)[60]. The evidence, though, is that a blood pressure of <120/75mmHg is ideal for renal protection, and recent recommendations from a number of professional bodies have suggested this lower target. It is highly unlikely that these very strict targets will be achieved by use of a single antihypertensive agent; most patients will need two or more antihypertensive agents from different drug classes.

In type 2 diabetes the first-line renoprotective therapy should be an ARB, as this class of agents has the strongest evidence base and is generally extremely well tolerated. An ACE inhibitor is an alternative, but less well proven, treatment. Beyond this, most patients will require a second, third or even fourth antihypertensive agent from different drug classes to achieve their target blood pressures. Combination of an ACE inhibitor with an ARB has been shown in preliminary studies to have an additive effect in reducing both blood pressure and urinary protein excretion, but further information on this is awaited from large trials with more specific endpoints.

It is the author's practice to use a thiazide or thiazide-like diuretic as a second-line antihypertensive agent. The advantages of thiazides are that they combine extremely well with inhibitors of the RAS, are inexpensive and have established safety profiles. They have also been shown to confer cardiovascular protection in the general population with hypertension, with reductions in the incidence of stroke, heart failure and cardiovascular disease[32]. Thiazide-like diuretics such as indapamide exert similar effects but appear to have better metabolic side-effect profiles and are preferred in some quarters[61].

Third-line agents can include β-blockers. These drugs are relatively inexpensive and effective in lowering blood pressure. They have also been shown to confer a degree of cardiovascular protection, particularly following a myocardial infarction[32]. There are, however, problems with tolerability and a high rate of side effects, including metabolic disturbances, erectile dysfunction and reduced warning symptoms of hypoglycaemia, although the latter is almost certainly over-estimated. The β-blockers clearly have a role when there is coincident hypertension and angina. Otherwise, the author does not commonly use them, except in more resistant cases of hypertension.

Alternative agents include CCBs such as amlodipine or felodipine[32]. They are suitable for once-daily dosing, relatively inexpensive, efficacious in lowering blood pressure and, again, have shown evidence of cardioprotective properties. CCBs are metabolically neutral and have a relatively good safety profile, although they are associated with a high incidence of minor side effects such as facial flushing and ankle oedema. They are suitable agents to use in the management of hypertension in diabetes, but in the context of nephropathy the author would normally reserve them for third-line treatment.

Specific α-blockers such as doxazosin should only be used as part of combination treatment and not as first-line agents[32]. They are efficacious in lowering blood pressure, although there are no hard outcome data that would support their use as first-line therapy. The α-blockers are metabolically neutral and can work positively in combination with other agents.

Cardiovascular disease

Although attention to very strict blood pressure control is vital, it is worth remembering that the majority of these patients will die from cardiovascular disease before they die from uraemia! It is extremely important that they are given a 'full house' of cardio-protective therapies. This should encompass advice on diet and lifestyle, including the benefits of increased physical activity and, where relevant, reduction in alcohol consumption and cessation of cigarette smoking. Pharmacotherapy should also be provided, and not delayed in any way. It is the author's opinion that, since type 2 diabetes is a cardiovascular disease, all such patients should normally be prescribed a statin, probably together with low-dose aspirin. This is especially important in patients with both incipient and overt diabetic nephropathy, since the risk of cardiovascular mortality is so much greater than in normoalbuminuric patients.

Dyslipidaemia

Both the Heart Protection Study (HPS)[62] and the Collaborative AtoRvastatin Diabetes Study (CARDS)[63] showed very clearly the benefits of treating dyslipidaemia in patients with diabetes. The basic message from all of the trials with statins, in both the diabetic and the general populations, is that a 20% reduction in total serum cholesterol is associated with a reduction of around 30% in the relative risk of coronary heart disease.

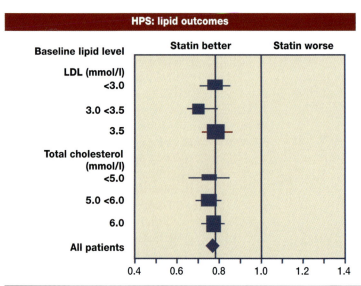

Fig 5.1 Cardiovascular risk reduction was the same at all levels of serum cholesterol in subjects given a fixed-dose statin in the HPS (adapted from Heart Protection Study Collaborative Group. *Lancet* 2002[61] with permission from Elsevier).

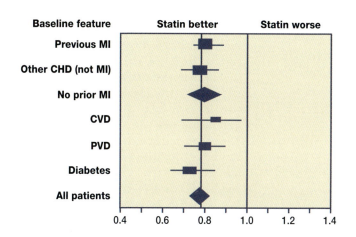

HPS: CHD outcomes

Fig 5.2 Reduced risk of all types of cardiovascular events in subjects given a fixed-dose statin in the HPS (adapted from Heart Protection Study Collaborative Group. *Lancet* 2002[61] with permission from Elsevier).

The HPS extended these findings further. It included over 20,000 patients, of whom almost 4,000 had diabetes but no clinically evident cardiovascular disease. The age range was up to 80 years and the lower limit for total cholesterol for entry into the trial was 3.5mmol/l. All patients received a fixed dose of 40mg simvastatin with no titration against serum cholesterol. Over five years there was a relative risk reduction in coronary heart disease of approximately 30% in both diabetic and non-diabetic subjects. Importantly, the same relative risk reduction was seen at all levels of serum cholesterol and in all ages up to 80 years (Fig 5.1). There were also reductions in the risk of stroke, transient ischaemic attack and peripheral vascular disease (Fig 5.2). Thus, no lower limit below which no benefit is derived from the use of statins has been determined. All patients with a high cardiovascular risk (which includes not only those with diabetic nephropathy, but all individuals with diabetes) are at sufficiently high risk that they should be started on a statin at any level of total cholesterol above 3.5mmol/l.

This contention is supported by the results of CARDS, which recruited 3,000 patients with type 2 diabetes and at least one other risk factor, but no history of coronary heart disease[63]. The subjects, who were drawn from 132 sites in the UK and Ireland, were randomised to receive either atorvastatin 10mg once daily or placebo, with a minimum follow-up period of four years. The primary endpoint was time to first major cardiac event (coronary heart disease, death, non-fatal myocardial infarction, revascularisation, unstable angina, stroke or resuscitated cardiac arrest). This study demonstrated dramatic risk reductions in cardiovascular events and mortality in subjects given atorvastatin (Fig 5.3).

Assessing risk

The message that emerges from both HPS and CARDS is that the concept of primary prevention in type 2 diabetes is redundant. It has been shown very clearly that a patient with diabetes who has never had a cardiovascular event is at as high a risk of such an event as a non-diabetic patient who has previously had a cardiovascular event[13]. Both HPS and CARDS have shown that intervention with statin therapy should not be determined by levels of serum cholesterol alone and, indeed, the same relative benefit is shown at all levels of cholesterol.

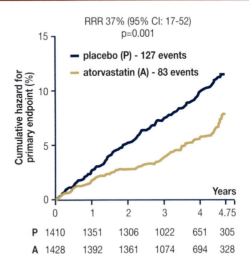

Fig 5.3 Dramatic risk reductions in primary cardiovascular endpoint (time to first serious cardiac event) in patients with type 2 diabetes given a statin (atorvastatin) in the CARDS study (adapted from Colhoun et al. *Lancet* 2004[62] with permission from Elsevier).

Despite these data, present recommendations from NICE (National Institute for Health and Clinical Excellence) state that, in order to receive a statin, a patient with diabetes should have a 10-year risk of coronary heart disease of >15%[64]. This allows for around 70% of patients with diabetes to be prescribed a statin – but what about the remaining 30%? Unfortunately, practitioners may find themselves in the situation of having a relatively young patient with type 2 diabetes whose 10-year coronary heart disease risk is predicted to be <15%, using the Framingham risk equation. The reason for this is that the equation does not adjust for age and does not take into account proteinuria (which, as stated above, is a very ominous finding associated with very high cardiovascular risk), racial origin or degree of glycaemia. It is the author's opinion that such cardiovascular risk equations should not be used in patients with diabetes, and this view is supported by the recent British Hypertension Society guidelines, which recommend that all patients with diabetes, particularly those with incipient or overt nephropathy, should be given a statin[60].

This argument applies equally to the case for low-dose aspirin in these patients, as shown by the results of the HOT study[36]. Individuals with incipient and overt nephropathy are at such high cardiovascular risk that they should routinely be offered low-dose (75mg daily) aspirin. If there are problems with tolerability or contraindications to aspirin, clopidogrel is a suitable alternative.

The importance of glycaemic control

It is perhaps surprising that a diabetes specialist has hardly mentioned glucose in this small book! Good glycaemic control will help to prevent the development of nephropathy, but there is little evidence that, once nephropathy is established, glycaemic control will prevent further progression. Having said this, there are a host of reasons to try and maintain optimum glycaemic control, including the general wellbeing of the patient and prevention of other vascular complications. It would also seem reasonable to assume, although we do not have absolute evidence, that some benefit will accrue from improvement in glycaemic control in terms of slowing the progression of nephropathy.

Glycaemic control can be difficult to achieve in patients who are in the more advanced stages of nephropathy, and most will require insulin. For those with type 2 diabetes and incipient or overt nephropathy, but no evidence of significant renal impairment, metformin remains the first-line oral antidiabetic treatment[65].

If adequate glycaemic control is not achieved with metformin, it can be combined with a sulphonylurea and/or a glitazone. In patients whose creatinine exceeds 150μmol/l (and some would say >130μmol/l), metformin should be avoided because of the increased risk of development of the extremely rare (but very serious) complication of lactic acidosis[65].

If glycaemic targets are still not met, insulin treatment should be considered, particularly as the diabetes becomes more advanced. Many patients manage with an oral agent combined with a basal insulin, and this regimen has the advantages of simplicity and general acceptability. With further deterioration in control, however, more intensive insulin regimens may be required, such as additional bolus injections of rapid-acting insulin before each meal or, alternatively, twice- or thrice-daily pre-mixed insulins. It is beyond the scope of this book to consider these in any detail.

KEY LEARNING POINTS

Given that type 2 diabetes is a cardiovascular disease, the concept of primary prevention is redundant and there is therefore no need to use cardiovascular risk tables

Patients with type 2 diabetes are generally at such high cardiovascular risk that they should normally be taking a statin and low-dose aspirin. This applies particularly in the context of incipient and overt nephropathy, where risk tables will dramatically underestimate the true risk!

All patients with incipient or overt nephropathy should be given antihypertensive treatment that includes an inhibitor of the renin angiotensin system

Good glycaemic control, commonly requiring the use of insulin injections, is also important in reducing the likelihood of renal damage and other vascular complications, and for general wellbeing

6 Multiprofessional management

Diabetic renal disease is a potentially devastating complication. As the prevalence of diabetes increases (particularly type 2 diabetes), we are likely to see a commensurate increase in the number of patients with renal complications. Indeed, as illustrated in Chapter 1, the number of patients entering end-stage renal disease in Europe is increasing in an exponential fashion. It should be pointed out, however, that one of the reasons for this massive increase in the number of patients developing renal disease is quite simply the fact that we now have the drugs to reduce their risk of dying from cardiovascular disease.

Primary care: prevention, screening and management of incipient renal disease

In the UK, most patients with type 2 diabetes are managed in primary care. The new General Medical Services contract for primary care physicians includes a requirement for annual screening for the presence of microalbuminuria in patients with type 2 diabetes; unfortunately, this target does not carry many points! Thus, there may be less incentive for general practices to perform this screening test when compared with others. However, the finding of microalbuminuria defines an extremely high-risk group of patients who may go on to develop overt nephropathy. It is, therefore, incumbent on primary care physicians to ensure that all of these patients have an annual review that includes screening for evidence of incipient nephropathy. In addition, dipstick testing for proteinuria should be carried out at each clinic visit. Once overt proteinuria has developed, it is much more difficult to intervene to prevent further disease progression.

In general practice, the multiprofessional team usually consists of the GP, the practice nurse and, where required, the dietitian and the community podiatrist. Measures such as blood pressure assessment and testing for albuminuria, as well as sending off blood tests, are normally the responsibility of the practice nurse, who needs to be both confident and competent in his or her tasks. Assessment for nephropathy must include both dipstick testing and measurement of blood pressure.

A finding of hypertension and proteinuria in a patient with type 2 diabetes has to be treated seriously. As discussed earlier in this book, these patients need to be identified for very rapid and aggressive management to achieve blood pressure control, normally using combinations of antihypertensive agents from different drug classes, and almost always including an inhibitor of the RAS. They should also routinely be prescribed a statin and low-dose aspirin. Particular attention to glycaemic control is advised and many of these patients will require insulin.

Secondary care: management of chronic hypertension and overt renal disease

A number of primary care trusts now have joint protocols agreed with secondary care colleagues for the management of diabetic renal disease. There comes a point when many of these patients need to be seen in secondary care, ideally in a diabetes/renal clinic. Certainly, where blood pressure targets are not being achieved in a patient with incipient nephropathy, he or she should be seen in secondary care. It is also important to appreciate that one complication is often associated with others. *Most patients who have nephropathy will also have (often advanced) retinopathy, and many will have evidence of cardiovascular disease.*

Once proteinuria becomes overt, patients should be assessed in secondary care. In our service, we provide a weekly diabetes/renal clinic and patients can be seen and assessed by both the diabetologist and the nephrologist. During that assessment they also have the advantage of being seen, as required, by the diabetes specialist nurse and the dietitian. Management plans are developed in collaboration with the patient and his or her primary care physician. The most important aspect of management remains strict blood pressure control and attention to other cardiovascular risk factors. Once assessed, some of these patients can be returned to primary care, but others will need very careful follow-up, particularly where there is deteriorating renal function.

If renal function does deteriorate, other complications may come into play, such as increased frequency of anaemia. Such patients may need the benefit of erythropoietin injections and consideration for dialysis. This is where the secondary care multiprofessional team is important, with the patient seeing not only the nephrologist but also the renal dialysis nurses. Dialysis is best instituted at a relatively early stage in view of the rapid progression of renal disease often seen in patients with diabetes. There is also an increased risk of problems such as sepsis, difficulties with access sites and cardiovascular events in those with diabetes. They require very careful management and this is a highly specialised area. Further discussion of dialysis programmes and renal transplantation is beyond the scope of this book.

It should be emphasised, however, that outcomes for patients undergoing dialysis for diabetic renal disease are less certain than those in the general population with chronic renal failure; this applies even more in the case of transplantation. The important point, therefore, is to identify these patients early and prevent them ever getting near a dialysis machine!

KEY LEARNING POINTS

All patients with diabetes should be screened at each visit for overt proteinuria and, if absent, should be assessed for the presence of microalbuminuria at least annually

All patients with incipient nephropathy whose blood pressure targets are not being achieved, and all those with evidence of overt nephropathy, should be referred to secondary care

Most patients with diabetic renal disease will also have diabetic retinopathy, and many will have cardiovascular disease

Early identification of diabetic nephropathy is vital in order to prevent or slow progression to overt and, ultimately, end-stage renal disease

References

1. World Health Organization. The Diabetes Programme 2004 (www.who.int/diabetes/ent)
2. Wild S, Roglic G, Green A et al. Global prevalence of diabetes: estimates for the year 2000 and projections for 2030. *Diabetes Care* 2004; 27: 1047-53.
3. Office for Population Censuses and Surveys. *Health Survey for England*. London: HMSO, 1991.
4. Kuczmarski RJ, Flegal KM, Campbell SM et al. Increasing prevalence of overweight among US adults. The National Health and Nutrition Examination Surveys 1960 to 1991. *JAMA* 1994; 272: 205-11.
5. Colditz GA, Willett WC, Rotnitzky A et al. Weight gain as a risk factor for clinical diabetes mellitus in women. *Ann Intern Med* 1995; 122: 481-86.
6. Gortmaker SL, Must A, Sobol AM et al. Television viewing as a cause of increasing obesity among children in the United States, 1986-1990. *Arch Pediatr Adolesc Med* 1996; 150: 356-62.
7. Reilly JJ, Dorosty AR. Epidemic of obesity in UK children. *Lancet* 1999; 354: 1874-75.
8. Borch-Johnsen K, Andersen PK, Deckert T. The effect of proteinuria on relative mortality in type 1 (insulin-dependent) diabetes mellitus. *Diabetologia* 1985; 28: 590-96.
9. Diabetes care and research in Europe: the Saint Vincent Declaration. *Diabet Med* 1990; 7: 360.
10. Kannel WB, McGee, DL. Diabetes and cardiovascular risk factors: the Framingham study. *Circulation* 1979; 59: 8-13.
11. Fisher M, Shaw KM. Diabetes – a state of premature cardiovascular death. *Pract Diabet Int* 2001; 18: 183-84.
12. Stamler J, Vaccaro O, Neaton JD et al. Diabetes, other risk factors and 12-year mortality for men as screened in the multiple risk factor intervention trial. *Diabetes Care* 1993; 16: 434-44.
13. Haffner SM, Lehto S, Ronnemaa T et al. Mortality from coronary heart disease in subjects with type 2 diabetes and in non-diabetic subjects with and without prior myocardial infarction. *N Engl J Med* 1998; 339: 229-34.
14. Anderson AR, Christiansen JS, Anderson JK et al. Diabetic nephropathy in type 1 (insulin-dependent) diabetes: an epidemiological study. *Diabetologia* 1983; 25: 496-501.
15. MacLeod JM, Lutale J, Marshall SM. Albumin excretion and vascular deaths in NIDDM. *Diabetologia* 1995; 38: 610-16.
16. Remuzzi G, Schieppati A, Ruggenenti P. Nephropathy in patients with type 2 diabetes. *N Engl J Med* 2002; 346: 1145-51.
17. Ritz E. Albuminuria and vascular damage – the vicious twins. *N Engl J Med* 2003; 348: 2349-52.
18. Gall MA, Hougaard P, Borch-Johnsen K et al. Risk factors for development of incipient and overt diabetic nephropathy in patients with non-insulin dependent diabetes mellitus: prospective, observational study. *Br Med J* 1997; 314: 783-88.
19. Adler AI, Stevens RJ, Manley SE, et al. Development and progression of nephropathy in type 2 diabetes: the United Kingdom Prospective Diabetes Study (UKPDS 64). *Kidney Int* 2003; 63: 225-32.
20. United Kingdom Prospective Diabetes Study (UKPDS) Group. Intensive blood glucose control with sulphonylureas or insulin compared with conventional treatment and risk of complications in patients with type 2 diabetes (UKPDS 33). *Lancet* 1998; 352: 837-53.
21. Mogensen CE. Microalbuminuria predicts clinical proteinuria and early mortality in maturity-onset diabetes. *N Engl J Med* 1984; 310: 356-60.
22. Nelson RG, Knowler WC, Pettitt DJ et al. Assessing risk of overt nephropathy in diabetic patients from albumin excretion in untimed urine specimens. *Arch Intern Med* 1991; 151: 1761-65.
23. Jarrett RJ, Alberti GC, Argyropoulos A et al. Microalbuminuria predicts mortality in non-insulin-dependent diabetics. *Diabet Med* 1984; 1: 17-19.
24. Lacourcière Y, Belanger A, Godin C et al. Long-term comparison of losartan and enalapril on kidney function in hypertensive type 2 diabetics with early nephropathy. *Kidney Int* 2000; 58: 762-69.
25. Valmadrid CT, Kleine R, Moss SE et al. The risk of cardiovascular disease mortality associated with microalbuminuria and gross proteinuria in persons with older onset diabetes mellitus. *Arch Intern Med* 2000; 160: 1093-100.
26. International Diabetes Federation. The kidney issue. *Diabetes Voice* 2003; 48: Special Issue.
27. O'Donnell MJ, Chowdhury TA. Hypertension and nephropathy in diabetes. In: Barnett AH, Dodson PM

(eds). *Hypertension and Diabetes (3rd edn)*. London: Science Press, 2000; 21-31.

28. Barnett AH. Hypertension as a risk factor for diabetic vascular disease. In: Barnett AH, Dodson PM (eds). *Hypertension and Diabetes (3rd edn)*. London: Science Press, 2000; 11-20.

29. Ramsay L, Williams B, Johnston G et al. Guidelines for management of hypertension: report of the third working party of the British Hypertension Society. *J Human Hypertens* 1999; 13: 569-92.

30. Reaven GM. Role of insulin resistance in human disease [Banting Lecture]. *Diabetes* 1988; 37: 1595-1607.

31. Barnett AH. Pharmacology of antihypertensive drugs. In: Barnett AH, Dodson PM (eds). *Hypertension and Diabetes (3rd edn)*. London: Science Press, 2000; 33-42.

32. Drury PL, Smith GM, Ferris JB. Increased vasopressor responsiveness to angiotensin II in type 1 (insulin-dependent) diabetic patients without nephropathy. *Diabetologia* 1984; 27: 174-79.

33. Zatz R, Dunn BR, Meyer TW et al. Prevention of diabetic glomerulopathy in pharmacological amelioration of glomerular capillary hypertension. *J Clin Invest* 1986; 77: 1925-30.

34. The effect of intensive treatment of diabetes on the development and progression of long-term complications in insulin-dependent diabetes mellitus. The Diabetes Control and Complications Trial Research Group. *N Engl J Med* 1993; 329: 977-86.

35. Tight blood pressure control and risk of macrovascular and microvascular complications in type 2 diabetes: UKPDS 38. UK Prospective Diabetes Study Group. *Br Med J* 1998; 317: 703-13.

36. Hansson L, Zanchetti A, Carruthers SG et al. Effect of intensive blood-pressure lowering and low-dose aspirin in patients with hypertension: principal results of the Hypertension Optimal Treatment (HOT) randomised trial. HOT Study Group. *Lancet* 1998; 351: 1755-62.

37. Curb JD, Pressel SL, Cutler JA et al. Effect of diuretic-based antihypertensive treatment on cardiovascular disease risk in older diabetic patients with isolated systolic hypertension. Systolic Hypertension in the Elderly Program Cooperative Research Group. *JAMA* 1996; 276: 1886-92.

38. Tuomilehto J, Rastenyte D, Birkenhager WH et al. Effects of calcium-channel blockade in older patients with diabetes and systolic hypertension. Systolic Hypertension in Europe Trial Investigators. *N Engl J Med* 1999; 340: 677-84.

39. Hansson L, Lindholm LH, Niskanen L et al. Effect of angiotensin-converting-enzyme inhibition compared with conventional therapy on cardiovascular morbidity and mortality in hypertension: the Captopril Prevention Project (CAPPP) randomised trial. *Lancet* 1999; 353: 611-16.

40. Effects of ramipril on cardiovascular and micro-vascular outcomes in people with diabetes mellitus: results of the HOPE study and MICRO-HOPE substudy. Heart Outcomes Prevention Evaluation Study Investigators. *Lancet* 2000; 355: 253-59.

41. Barnett AH, Bain SC, Bouter P et al; Diabetics Exposed to Telmisartan and Enalapril Study Group. Angiotensin-receptor blockade versus converting-enzyme inhibition in type 2 diabetes and nephropathy. *N Engl J Med* 2004; 351: 1952-61.

42. Christensen CK, Mogensen CE. Effect of antihypertensive treatment on the progression of incipient diabetic nephropathy. *Hypertension* 1985; 7 (Suppl 2): 109-13.

43. Agardh CD, Garcia-Puig J, Charbonnel B et al. Greater reduction of urinary albumin excretion in hypertensive type II diabetic patients with incipient nephropathy by lisinopril than by nifedipine. *J Human Hypertens* 1996; 10: 185-92.

44. Lewis EJ, Hunsicker LG, Bain RP et al. The effect of angiotensin-converting-enzyme inhibition on diabetic nephropathy. The Collaborative Study Group. *N Engl J Med* 1993; 329: 1456-62.

45. Ruggenenti P, Fassi A, Ilieva AP et al. Preventing microalbuminuria in type 2 diabetes. *N Engl J Med* 2004; 351: 1941-51.

46. Dahlof B, Devereux RB, Kjeldsen SE et al. Cardiovascular morbidity and mortality in the Losartan Intervention For Endpoint reduction in hypertension study (LIFE): a randomised trial against atenolol. *Lancet* 2002; 359: 995-1003.

47. Pfeffer MA, Swedberg K, Granger CB et al; CHARM Investigators and Committees. Effects of candesartan on mortality and morbidity in patients with chronic heart failure: the CHARM-Overall programme. *Lancet* 2003; 362: 759-66.

48. McMurray JJ, Ostergren J, Swedberg K et al; CHARM Investigators and Committees. Effects of candesartan in patients with chronic heart failure and reduced left-ventricular systolic function taking angiotensin-converting-enzyme inhibitors: the CHARM-Added trial. *Lancet* 2003; 362: 767-71.

49. Granger CB, McMurray JJ, Yusuf S et al; CHARM Investigators and Committees. Effects of candesartan in patients with chronic heart failure and reduced left-ventricular systolic function intolerant to angiotensin-converting-enzyme inhibitors: the CHARM-Alternative trial. *Lancet* 2003; 362: 772-76.

50. Yusuf S, Pfeffer MA, Swedberg K et al; CHARM Investigators and Committees. Effects of candesartan in patients with chronic heart failure and preserved left-ventricular ejection fraction: the CHARM-Preserved trial. *Lancet* 2003; 362: 777-81.

51. White HD. Candesartan and heart failure: the allure of CHARM [commentary]. *Lancet* 2003; 362: 754-55.

52. Parving H-H, Lehnert H, Brochner-Mortensen J et al; Irbesartan in Patients with Type 2 Diabetes and Microalbuminuria Study Group. The effect of irbesartan on the development of diabetic nephropathy in patients with type 2 diabetes. *N Engl J Med* 2001; 345: 870-78.

53. Lewis EJ, Hunsicker LG, Clarke WR et al. Collaborative Study Group. Renoprotective effect of the angiotensin-receptor antagonist irbesartan in patients with nephropathy due to type 2 diabetes. *N Engl J Med* 2001; 345: 851-60.

54. Brenner BM, Cooper ME, de Zeeuw D et al. RENAAL Study Investigators. Effect of losartan on renal and cardiovascular outcomes in patients with type 2 diabetes and nephropathy. *N Engl J Med* 2001; 345: 861-69.

55. Lacourcière Y, Belanger A, Godin C et al. Long-term comparison of losartan and enalapril on kidney function in hypertensive type 2 diabetics with early nephropathy. *Kidney Int* 2000; 58: 762-69.

56. Pitt B, Poole-Wilson A, Segal R et al. Effect of losartan compared with captopril on mortality in patients with symptomatic heart failure: randomised trial – the Losartan Heart Failure Survival Study ELITE II. *Lancet* 2000; 355: 1582-87.

57. Dickstein K, Kjekshus J; OPTIMAAL Steering Committee of the OPTIMAAL Study Group. Effects of losartan and captopril on mortality and morbidity in high-risk patients after acute myocardial infarction: the OPTIMAAL randomised trial. Optimal Trial in Myocardial Infarction with Angiotensin II Antagonist Losartan. *Lancet* 2002; 360: 752-60.

58. Pfeffer MA, McMurray JJV, Velazquez EJ et al. Valsartan, captopril, or both in myocardial infarction complicated by heart failure, left ventricular dysfunction, or both. *N Engl J Med* 2003; 349: 1893-906. [Erratum, *N Engl J Med* 2004; 350: 203.]

59. Mogensen CE. Intervention strategies for microalbuminuria: the role of angiotensin II antagonists, including dual blockade with an ACE-I and a receptor blocker [abstract]. Third International Symposium on Angiotensin II Antagonism. London: UK 2000: A7.4

60. Williams B, Poulter NR, Brown KJ et al. Guidelines for management of hypertension: report of the fourth working party of the British Hypertension Society, 2004 – BHS IV. *J Human Hypertens* 2004; 18: 139-85.

61. Leonetti G, Emeriau JP, Knauf H et al. Evaluation of long-term efficacy of indapamide SR 1.5mg in elderly hypertensive patients. *Am J Hypertens* 2001; 14.4 (Suppl 1): A102-03.

62. Heart Protection Study Collaborative Group. MRC/BHF Heart Protection Study of cholesterol lowering with simvastain in 20,536 high-risk individuals: a randomised placebo-controlled trial. *Lancet* 2002; 360: 7-22.

63. Colhoun HM, Betteridge DJ, Durrington PN et al; CARDS Investigators. Primary prevention of cardiovascular disease with atorvastatin in type 2 diabetes in the Collaborative Atorvastatin Diabetes Study (CARDS): multicentre randomised placebo-controlled trial. *Lancet* 2004; 364: 685-96.

64. National Institute for Health and Clinical Excellence (NICE). *Management of Type 2 Diabetes – management of blood pressure and blood lipids. (Guideline H).* London: NICE, 2002.

65. Bailey CJ. Antidiabetic drugs. *Br J Cardiol* 2000; 7: 350-60.

Index